Fitness Lifestyle

Top 20 Fitness Lifestyle Tips to Get in Shape

By
Bring on Fitness

information contained within this document, including, but not limited to, errors, omissions, or inaccuracies.

About Bring On Fitness

Our passion for fitness gave life to **Bring On Fitness**. We started with the goal of helping as many people as we can. To educate, motivate and to help change peoples lives for the better. Bring On Fitness is not only for the fitness enthusiasts, but also for the beginner. We strongly believe nothing is more important than learning the basics and creating a strong foundation in both nutrition - through meal planning, and in exercise - by following a specific plan. This is just as important for the beginner, as it is for the experienced athlete.

We set high standards for ourselves, the information we share, and the products we carry. Our goal is to provide you with exceptional products that suit your needs and the knowledge and motivation to help you work towards and achieve your health and fitness goals.

Check us out at www.bringonfitness.com

"Our Mission is to have a positive impact in changing peoples lives. We will deliver the best possible fitness and nutrition solutions that will empower people to achieve their health and fitness goals."

Table of Contents

Introduction

Thank you for purchasing this book, *"Fitness Lifestyle – Top 20 Fitness Lifestyle Tips to Get in Shape."*

Do you want to get in shape and achieve your fitness and weight loss goals? I'm sure the answer is quite simply yes. To get fit you don't have to follow a crazy crash diet or anything of that sort. You merely have to make a couple of changes to your lifestyle. Your lifestyle dictates different aspects of your life, and if you can tweak it a little, you can achieve your goals.

In this book, you will learn about different fitness lifestyle tips that will help you to turn your life around. So, why don't we get started now?

I want to thank you once again for choosing this book, and I hope it brings you value!

Fitness Lifestyle Tips to Get in Shape

What does the phrase "a healthy lifestyle" mean? It means having a healthy body, which not only looks good but feels good as well. A healthy person will try to follow a healthy diet, maintain a healthy weight, and will exercise regularly.

Do you want to lead a healthy life? Then read along; you will learn about different lifestyle tips that will help you lead a healthy life. Moreover, you can lose weight while you improve your overall health.

Tip #1: The Weight Loss Equation

The simplest way to define the weight loss equation is the point where you start to lose weight. You will lose weight when your calorie consumption is lower than the calories your body burns. So the idea is to induce your body into a state of calorie deficit.

As a rule of thumb, one pound of fat is approximately equivalent to 3500 calories. When your body reaches a calorie deficit of 3500 calories, you will lose one pound of fat! It means that you have to monitor the calories you consume daily. It doesn't mean that you have to obsess over every calorie you consume. Just be mindful of what you eat! There are various apps that you can use to monitor your calorie intake. Another alternative is to maintain a food journal.

Tip #2: Predefined Hours

Irregular eating habits can wreak havoc on your overall health. Create a schedule for yourself, and stick to it. Try to eat at the same time daily. When you create an eating schedule for yourself, your biological clock syncs your brain and stomach. It might sound weird, but it helps.

When you eat at predefined hours, your food cravings will reduce. Your body gets used to eating at a particular time daily, and it won't deviate from it. So the urge to snack on a bag of chips or gobble down a pint of ice cream will reduce and eventually stop. Not just that, but it also provides your body with sufficient time to digest the food you eat. Better digestion leads to better absorption of food in your body. All this helps to improve your energy levels.

Tip #3: Stay Hydrated

It is incredibly important to drink plenty of water. How many glasses of water do you drink per day? You probably have six glasses of water. Well, that doesn't cut it, and your body needs at least eight glasses of water daily. Lack of water makes you dehydrated, causes tiredness, and even dries up your skin. If you don't want any premature wrinkles and want your skin to retain its sheen and glow, you should drink plenty of water. You can jazz up regular water by adding a couple of sprigs of mint and slices of lemon to it. Detox water is a great idea, and it does help to flush out all the toxins from your body.

Drinking plenty of water also aids in weight loss. Water makes you feel full, thereby effectively curbing hunger. You can start your day with a glass of water! Always carry a water bottle with you, and drink a glass of water before every meal. Water has zero calories and plenty of health benefits.

Tip #4: Don't Follow Crazy Diets

It is essential not just to lose weight but to keep it off as well. Therefore, you should follow a diet that will work for you in the long run. So you shouldn't follow any crazy crash diets that provide short-term results. You might be able to lose a couple of pounds with a crash diet, but when you stop the diet, all the weight you lost will pile on rather quickly.

Instead, you should learn to lose weight safely. If you are new to the world of dieting, then you might not know where you should start. Before you select a diet, make sure that you can follow it in the long run as well. So take some time and do plenty of research.

If you want a weight loss regime that is sustainable in the long run, then you should eat healthily and exercise regularly. You can shed a couple of pounds by cutting out major food groups from your daily diet, but it isn't sustainable in the long run. If you want your body to function optimally, it needs all the major food groups.

When you find a diet that works well for you, make sure that it's the only diet you follow. Don't follow two or more diets together. You will primarily set yourself up for failure by doing so. If you suffer from any health conditions, always consult your physician before you start the diet.

Tip #5: Select Foods Wisely

Even if you don't follow a diet in a formal sense, you should be selective about the type of foods you eat. If you want to lose weight, then you should learn to select your foods wisely. Having a well-balanced meal is essential. You have to make sure that your body gets all the macros it needs. Load up half of your plate with vegetables and the other half with protein-rich food.

A balanced diet is rich in essential vitamins, minerals and nutrients while it is low in unnecessary fats and sugars. Make sure that you include the following food groups into your daily diet:

Protein

Focus on lean meats, such as lean cuts of chicken, fish, pork, lamb or beef. It is better to de-skin the meat, and always get rid of the unnecessary fats. Include a handful of nuts in your diet. Nuts have a high protein content, and they are great for a simple and easy snack as well. Dairy products are also an option as they are full of calcium, healthy fats, and Vitamin D.

Vegetables

Vegetables are rich in vitamins and minerals. Green leafy vegetables are quite nutritious and are full of fiber. So be sure to include some greens in all your meals. You can also include a variety of plant-based protein as well. Plant-based proteins include soy products and a variety of lentils.

Fruits

Fruits are full of nutrients, and they make for an excellent snack. Try to opt for whatever fruit is in season. There is nothing better than seasonal produce. Fruits have natural sugars, but as long as you have them in reasonable quantities, it is right for you. If you want to control your sugar intake, then you should stay away from extremely sugary fruits like mangoes. If you're going to regulate your carb intake, then you should include avocados and melons.

Whole Grains

Always opt for whole grains instead of refined flours and grains.

Tip #6: Portions Matter

You should keep an eye on the portions you eat. It also helps to make sure that you have a well-balanced meal.

Your calorie intake shouldn't exceed the calories your body burns. If it does, then your body will just store all the excess calories you consume in the form of fat cells, and this leads to weight gain.

You don't have to use a measuring cup or a measuring scale to size your potions. You can measure them with your hand, and it is quite simple. Your palm signifies the size of protein you should consume. The recommended size of meat for a meal is about 3 ounces or the size and weight of a deck of cards. Your palm is just about the ideal size. The portion of veggies you should consume is equivalent to a clenched fist. Just cup your hand, and that's the number of carbs you should eat.

A fistful of carbs is the ideal size for a meal, and it can include rice, pasta, bread, or any other starchy vegetable. The portion of fats per meal should be equivalent to the size of your thumb. That's equivalent to a tablespoon. If you want to measure the proportion of cheese, then you can use your fingers. A serving of cheese should be approximately equal to two of your fingers. So, to sum it all up, you should have a piece of meat that fits into your palm, a fistful of veggies, and a cupped handful of carbs. Your thumb represents the portion of fats, and fingers will represent the portion of cheese. So the key to a balanced meal is quite literally in your hand.

While you eat, if you like to add extra salt to your food, you should stop doing that. Try to reduce your overall salt intake. Don't reach for the saltshaker when you eat a salad or have some fries. Excess sodium isn't good for your body, and it increases your blood pressure. Not just that, but it also increases the stress your heart experiences as well. It can also put unnecessary strain on your kidneys and hinder their performance. There are different flavoring agents that you can use instead of salt. Use spices to flavor your food, and opt for rock salt instead of refined salt.

Tip #7: No Sugary Drinks

It is okay to have a sugary drink once in a while, but not on a daily basis. Sodas are sugar laden, and regardless of how tempting they might be, they aren't good for your health. Consumption of excess sugar won't do your body any good.

They are full of preservatives, and they will wreak havoc on your overall health. If you reduce your soda and soft drink intake, you can save yourself the trouble of high blood sugar levels, clogged arteries, and unnecessary caffeine. Instead of sodas, you can have some lemonade. Have iced tea instead of cola. All aerated, sugary, and processed drinks will hurt your oral health!

If you want to shed those extra pounds, then it is a good idea to stay away from soda, but it is not just sodas that you should be mindful of. You should keep an eye out on your alcohol intake as well. It is perfectly all right to have a glass of wine or a pint of beer once in a while. However, if you consume alcohol regularly, it won't do your health any good. Did you know that there are plenty of carbs in alcohol that lead to unnecessary weight gain, especially in the abdominal region? If you reduce your alcohol intake, you can reduce your cholesterol levels as well.

It helps to increase HDL levels while reducing LDL levels. You might not understand this, but it is important to maintain the health of your heart. It improves your blood pressure levels as well. Apart from that, you can sleep better at night if you reduce or stop your intake of alcohol. When you get a good night's rest, you will automatically feel refreshed and energetic on the following day. When your body gets sufficient rest, you can function optimally. When you can function optimally, your overall productivity will improve.

An occasional glass of wine or a peg of whiskey is okay, but don't make it a habit. The perfect replacement for alcohol or alcoholic drinks would be water (sparkling or still), tea, or occasionally coffee. If you want to have some alcoholic beverage, then opt for champagne, dry wine, or spirits. Be mindful of the quantity you drink; those carbs can creep in at any time.

Tip #8: Patience Matters

You need to learn to be patient. You cannot expect to see a change overnight. It takes a while to form positive habits, and it isn't an easy process. Change isn't easy, but it is necessary for growth.

Be patient with yourself, and don't give up on your healthy lifestyle. All good things take time, and the results will certainly be worth your while. You can see a positive change in your body within two weeks if you stick to a healthy diet and exercise regularly. If it feels like your weight loss has come to a standstill, then you should slightly tweak your diet. It is all about trial and error until you find a diet that works perfectly well for you.

Remember that Rome wasn't built in a day! If you lose patience, you will get frustrated and will revert to old ways. At times, you can indulge in a couple of cheat days. Don't feel guilty for what you eat. If you break your diet knowingly, then treat it as an isolated incident. Don't beat yourself up over it, and don't be too hard on yourself.

Tip #9: Morning Routine

Having a proper morning routine is imperative. Instead of staying up late at night, it makes sense to wake up early in the morning. Always start your day with a hearty breakfast. Breakfast is the most important meal of the day, and you shouldn't skip it. It is the most important meal of the day because it provides the necessary energy to keep going through the day.

Moreover, the best time to exercise is early in the morning! Create a morning routine for yourself. It will help to set the tone for the rest of the day. Reserve your morning hours to do something productive, and don't waste those precious hours. Put your gadgets away, don't check your email, but instead, sit down and have a healthy breakfast.

Tip #10: Exercise Buddy

If you find it difficult to exercise on your own, then you can find an exercise buddy to work out with you. You can team up with your spouse, friend, family member, or anyone else you want. Your exercise buddy will provide you with the necessary motivation to keep going even when you don't want to.

Not just that, but you will also be accountable to your buddy about whether you follow a healthy diet or not. It always helps to stay on track when you are accountable to someone else. So go ahead and find yourself an exercise buddy today!

Tip #11: Slow Down

Don't just gobble your food, and do learn to eat slowly. Did you know that your brain can take more than 20 minutes to register when the body feels full? So eat slowly, so that your brain can register when your stomach feels full. You can do this by following a straightforward technique that is known as the fork down. It is quite simple and will help you to enjoy your meal.

Start to eat smaller bites of food, and once you put the piece of food in your mouth, you have to place your fork on the plate. It can be a fork, spoon, chopsticks, or any other form of cutlery. The idea is to release your fork and not load it up with food while you still chew the food in your mouth. Let your hands be free while you chew. Don't prep your next bite before you swallow the current one. Now, you have to chew your food, and chew it well. Notice the different textures and flavors of food you eat. You should chew soft foods anywhere between 5 to 20 times before you swallow, and denser foods require you to chew about 30 times before you swallow. After you chew your food thoroughly, swallow it, and then you can pick up your fork again. Repeat this process whenever you eat, and it will help you to slow down while you eat. Not just that, but you will also become mindful of what you eat. It is important to savor what you eat, and you will also eat less than usual.

Tip #12: Don't Overeat

It is important to have well-balanced meals daily. You shouldn't skip any meals, but it doesn't mean that you should overeat. Eat only when you feel hungry, and don't eat otherwise.

Here are a couple of simple things you can do to avoid overeating: Learn to eat slowly. It isn't a new concept, but not many of us follow it. We are always in a rush these days. Take a moment, and slow down. Take a sip of water after every couple of bites, and chew your food thoroughly before you gulp it down.

Don't just mindlessly eat, and learn to enjoy the food you eat. Concentrate on the different textures, tastes, and flavors of the food you eat. Learn to savor every bite you eat, and make it an enjoyable experience. Make your first bite count, and let it satisfy your taste buds. Now is the time to let your inner gourmet chef out!

Use a smaller plate when you eat, and you can easily control your portions. Stay away from foods that are rich in calories and that won't satiate your hunger. Fill yourself up with foods that can satisfy your hunger and make you feel full for longer. If you have a big bowl of salad, you will feel fuller than you would if you have a small bag of chips. The calorie intake might be the same for both these things, but the hunger you will feel afterward differs. The idea is to fill yourself up with healthy foods before you think about junk food.

While you eat, make sure that you turn off all electronic gadgets. You tend to lose track of the food you eat while you watch TV.

Tip #13: Take a Walk during Lunch

Regardless of what your work is, you will get a lunch break daily. During your lunch break, make it a point to go out for a short stroll. It helps to get some fresh air. You will feel fresh and energized to go back to your work. Don't have a massive meal, as it will make you lethargic. You probably sit hunched over your laptop all day long, and a short walk is a perfect break your body and mind needs.

Tip #14: Different Mindset

Your mind is quite a brilliant thing. When you change your mindset toward a particular situation, it becomes better. If something seems difficult, break it down into smaller bits, and tackle them one thing at a time.

If you think that a diet is a pain, it will be painful to follow it. Instead, think of it as a means to achieve your goals, and it will become easier. It is all about your perspective on life. It is a classic case of "is the glass half-empty or half-full?" Create a positive mindset, and things will be more relaxed. This applies to all the aspects of your life and not just your diet. Make a list of reasons why you want to follow a healthy lifestyle. The next time you feel low on motivation, you can go through this list to feel better.

Tip #15: Make It Fun

Losing weight shouldn't feel like a chore. Exercise doesn't have to be boring and monotonous. You can make it fun! Make it a point to include at least 45 minutes of physical activity into your daily schedule.

You don't need a gym membership, and you don't have to run a marathon. Exercise doesn't mean sweating it out at the gym or lifting weights. There are different ways to exercise, and you don't necessarily have to go the gym. If you like to swim, you can swim for an hour on every alternate day. If you want to play a particular sport, you can play that sport daily. Even a leisurely stroll or jog will do.

There are plenty of alternatives to choose from! You can hike, dance, do yoga, or even Zumba. If you like any team sports, you can join a club. If you wish to watch TV, you can exercise while you watch your favorite sitcom. Place a treadmill or a stationary cycle in your living room, and exercise while you watch TV! If you like to walk, take a stroll at the mall. You can window shop while you exercise. If you like to dance, put on your dancing shoes, and join a dance class! Dance your way to weight loss and better health.

The idea is to make exercise more fun. If you do something you enjoy, it does get easy to stick to a schedule and do it regularly. Exercise assists in weight loss, burns fats, and strengthens your immune system as well. When you exercise, your body produces endorphins that help to elevate your mood.

Tip #16: Reduce Your Stress

Stress can make you forget about happiness. You should learn to manage stress efficiently and shouldn't let it complicate your life. Stress affects your health, hinders your ability to think, and even reduces your productivity. Therefore, it is essential to learn to manage your stress.

Stress can either make you overeat, or it can kill your appetite, and neither of these things is desirable if you want to lose weight and stay healthy.

Here are a couple of tips that will help you to manage stress effectively. Stay away from caffeine, nicotine, and alcohol as much as you can. These things aren't good for your health and will make you quite jittery. You might think that they help to calm you, but they have the opposite effect on your nervous system. They merely increase the stress you experience.

Stress stimulates your adrenaline glands and unnecessarily increases the supply of adrenaline in the body. Therefore, it is essential to engage in some form of physical exercise daily. It produces endorphins and helps to neutralize the harmful effects of too much adrenaline.

The best way to beat stress is to sleep. Make sure that you get sufficient sleep daily. When your body doesn't get adequate sleep, it becomes susceptible to stress. Give your body the time it needs to recharge itself. You can save yourself a lot of pressure by learning to say no. If you don't want to get burdened with unnecessary work, then all you need to do is say no. Another easy way to overcome stress is by talking it out. You can even maintain a stress journal.

Tip #17: Sufficient Sleep

Sufficient sleep is essential to maintaining your overall health. Not just that, but it also helps to elevate your mood and reduce the stress you feel.

Have you ever heard of the saying, "Early to bed, early to rise makes a man healthy, wealthy, and wise?" Well, this age-old saying is entirely correct. Your body needs about 7 hours of good quality sleep daily. If you cannot wake up on your own in the morning, you can set the alarm!

It isn't just about the number of hours you sleep, but the quality of sleep matters as well. You should create a sleep schedule for yourself, and follow it. Make it a point to go to bed at the same time every night. Sleep might not come quickly initially. However, after a while, it certainly does get easier. You can create a sleep time routine for yourself.

Don't have any caffeine or alcohol before you sleep as it disrupts sleep. Not just that, but don't have a massive meal either. Don't nap during the day, and include some physical activity.

Tip #18: Keep Track of Your Weight

Keeping track of your weight is essential. However, it doesn't mean that you should weigh yourself daily. Don't become obsessive about your weight. At times, you might not lose any weight, but your body might become toned. So measure your body, too!

Your weight will not stay constant, and it does fluctuate frequently. Certain things can affect your weight like any hormonal changes in your body, the recent meal you had, the exercises you do, and even the level of hydration. Your body weight fluctuates daily, and if you weigh yourself daily, it will not help. Weigh yourself once a week at the same time of day, and that's about it.

Tip #19: Avoid Exercise Mistakes

People who want to exercise to lose weight tend to make a critical mistake that prevents them from making the most of their exercise sessions. When you perform the same exercise repeatedly, at the same pace, and for the same duration, you won't lose any weight.

If you want to burn calories, then it is essential to speed up your heartbeat. Well, you can achieve this by gradually increasing the duration and pace of your exercises. The key is to push yourself continually. Vary your exercise routine. If you feel that a particular form of exercise seems to cause you discomfort, then you should consult a doctor immediately.

It is good to exercise on an empty stomach, but that doesn't mean you should starve yourself to lose weight. You should merely plan your day in such a manner that it allows you to exercise on an empty stomach. If you want to burn fat, then the best time to exercise is in the morning. If you're going to build muscle, then you should exercise in the afternoon or evening. Don't let your body run on fumes, as this just leads to exhaustion, and you can hurt yourself unknowingly.

Tip #20: Understand the Reason

Before you follow all the different tips discussed in this book, you should think about one thing. You should think about the reasons why you want to change your lifestyle.

You probably want to lead a healthier life, or lose weight, and a good diet is the first step toward getting there. If you do something without an aim or a reason, you will not get too far in life. Moreover, it helps you set specific goals for yourself. Goals help you to not only measure your progress, but also to see how far you have come.

You can tweak your diet and exercise program according to the development you make. However, make sure that you set realistic goals for yourself. Whenever you feel low on motivation, you can think about your reasons for following a healthy lifestyle. If that doesn't help, visualize a more robust and fitter version of yourself, and that will make you feel better.

Well, these steps aren't that difficult. Take some time out, and start including these tips into your daily life. You can start by adding one thing to your life at a time, and keep doing so until all the steps mentioned above have become a part of your life. You will undoubtedly see a positive change in your life in no time.

Conclusion

I would like to thank you once again for purchasing this book. I hope it proved to be an informative read.

It is quite easy to change your lifestyle. You don't have to do everything at once. You can start with one tip at a time! After a while, you won't have to make a conscious effort to follow these tips! Now, all that's left for you to do is get started, and follow the tips mentioned in this book.

Don't expect immediate changes overnight. It takes time, effort, patience and consistency to attain the results you desire. However, the effort you put in will provide you with excellent results! So make a plan, and take action to follow it.

Thank you, and remember to share how well these lifestyle tips work for you. You can do that here...

Thank you,

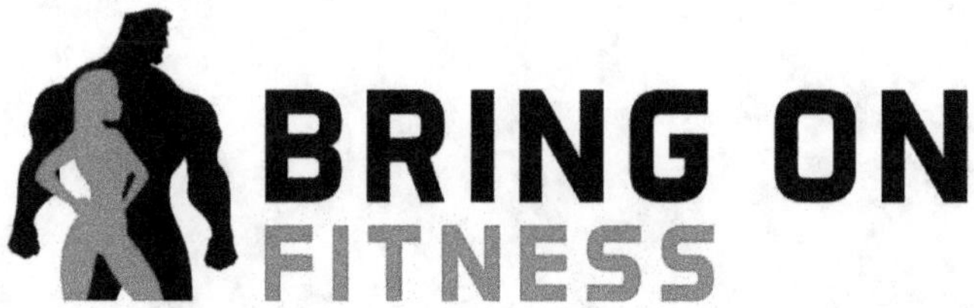

Resources

30

https://www.muscleandfitness.com/nutrition/lose-fat/20-tips-shed-body-fat-good-fast

https://www.verywellfit.com/simple-ways-to-live-a-healthy-lifestyle-1231193